Brain Injury

Living a Productive Life After a Stroke or Traumatic Brain Injury

By

Walter L. Kilcullen

ISBN-10: 1492116602
ISBN-13: 9781492116608

TABLE OF CONTENTS

Part III: Living a Productive Life after a Brain Injury

Part IV: Research and Recovery

INTRODUCTION

I had been a mentor for brain injury survivors for several years when I was sitting in the main lobby of Kessler Institute for Rehabilitation in New Jersey, waiting for one of my BIFs (brain injured friends), and saw something that reminded me of how complex the brain really is. A therapist was instructing a stroke survivor to circle around the perimeter of the room in her wheelchair. The patient was able to complete the task until she reached a spot about half way around where she turned into the center of the room. The therapist corrected her, but no matter how many times the task was attempted, the patient continued to turn in at the same spot. Every brain injury survivor has some disability, mild or extreme, or somewhere in between. But I am continually surprised when I see something like this with no explanation of why.

It seems that every month a new book comes out about stroke or traumatic brain injury, so I never thought about writing a book. I have been a staff writer for strokenetwork.org for the last two years and recently received an e-mail from a reader suggesting I write a book about making life better after a stroke or traumatic brain injury (TBI).

So my book focuses on how to live a better life after a stroke or brain injury. I have no medical degree and no background in treating brain injury. My background includes 22 years as a high school counselor and twelve years experience as a mentor for both acquired brain injury (stroke, aneurism, arteriovenous malformation, etc.) and traumatic brain injury (any external blow to the head that has caused the brain to be injured.)

About twelve years ago I heard that a woman I knew had a massive stroke and was in the hospital. When I went to see her, she could not talk (aphasia), and was paralyzed on her right side. I learned that her family was spread out in Florida, Texas, and California, so she did not have needed support from family. I started seeing her almost daily and became really interested in how the brain works. I found out about a training program offered by the Brain Injury Alliance of New Jersey to become a mentor. I went to the training and have been mentoring survivors ever since. I devote a chapter on mentoring so I won't describe what a mentor does now.

All but the first chapter of this book was published in the strokenetwork.org newsletter from July, 2009 to September, 2013, with permission from strokenetwork.org. The chapters, which were articles in the newsletters, were revised and updated where ever needed. Since it is a publication for stroke survivors, many of the studies throughout the book were or are stroke studies. In almost every case, however, the results apply to TBI survivors.

In a way, I did not really write this book myself because much of the book comes from interviewing neurologists, doctors, nurses, physical therapists, and other experts in the field. I include chapters on some basics such as risk factors for stroke, common brain injuries, how to avoid stroke and TBI, and chapters on specific results of a brain injury. Feel free to skip any of the topics that do not pertain to you.

And finally, I have written this book in simple language eliminating most of the technical terms so understanding is not difficult. But most importantly, some of the chapters are based on current research and I strongly urge the reader to follow ongoing and continuing research by going to web sites that I include with these chapters. This is especially important for chapters on stem cell research, new drugs being studied, transcranial magnetic stimulation research, and aphasia research.

Part I: Basics for Stroke and TBI

Chapter 1: Facts about Traumatic Brain Injury

The Center for Disease Control keeps statistics for TBI. The CDC states, "A Traumatic Brain Injury (TBI) is defined as a blow or jolt to the head or a penetrating head injury that disrupts the function of the brain."

Of the 1.7 million who sustain a TBI each year in the United States:

52,000 die

275,000 are hospitalized

1.365 million are treated and released at some point from a hospital

The leading causes of a TBI are:

Falls 35.2%

Motor vehicle accidents 17.3%

Assaults 10%

Unknown/other 21%

The CDC does not yet have statistics concerning military TBI, but the leading cause for active duty soldiers is blasts from an explosive device.

Only common sense suggestions can help prevent a TBI such as making sure carpeting is not lose to prevent falling; making sure that you do not drive carelessly; and wearing a helmet when riding a bicycle. Males are 1.5 times more likely than females to sustain a TBI. Two age groups at the highest risk for a TBI are 0 to 4 year olds and 15 to 19 year olds.

Chapter 2: Risk Factors for Stroke

Chances are that most readers of this chapter have had a stroke. The risk factors in this chapter, one or more of which have contributed to your stroke, carry the same risk factors in preventing a second stroke. Risk factors are different than causes. There are two basic causes of a stroke. First, is the formation of a clot that makes its way to an artery that blocks blood flow to the brain. This causes what we know as an *Ischemic Stroke.* The second cause, a result of bleeding in the brain, is a *Hemorrhagic Stroke.* (Approximately 87% of strokes are ischemic; 13% are hemorrhagic).

Most stroke survivors and even the general public know the primary risk factors for stroke. These include high blood pressure, high cholesterol, diabetes, and smoking. This chapter will look at all of these risk factors and secondary factors, some of which are too often overlooked.

High Blood Pressure: High blood pressure is the greatest risk factor for stroke. High BP puts unnecessary stress on blood vessels and arteries, causing them to thicken and deteriorate. When blood vessel walls thicken, substances such as cholesterol may break off and block an artery to the brain causing an ischemic stroke. High blood pressure can also put undue stress on a vessel or artery leading to a brain bleed and a hemorrhagic stroke.

High LDL Cholesterol: High cholesterol, which causes plaque build-up, can block normal blood flow to the brain and cause an ischemic stroke.

Atherosclerosis is the progressive build-up of cholesterol or other fatty deposits in the arteries that will eventually block flow to the brain causing a stroke.

Peripheral Arterial Disease (PAD): When plaque build-up from cholesterol clogs the arteries, it can also lead to the blockage of blood supply to the legs. This causes leg cramps and should be a warning that you may have atherosclerosis in other arteries.

<u>Diabetes:</u> Diabetes causes destructive changes in the blood vessels throughout the body, including the brain. Over time, high glucose levels damage nerve and blood vessels, leading to complications including stroke. The health risk of cardiovascular disease, including stroke, is two and a half times greater in people with diabetes compared to people without diabetes. Further, stroke is the leading cause of death among people with diabetes.

<u>Smoking:</u> The risk of stroke for smokers is between two and two and a half times that of non smokers. Studies have shown that smoking reduces the amount of oxygen in the blood, causing the heart to work harder and allowing blood clots to form more easily. Smoking also increases the amount of plaque in the arteries, which may block blood flow to the brain, causing a stroke.

<u>Atrial Fibrillation:</u> A person with A-Fib is five times more likely to have a stroke than someone without A-FIB. A-Fib is caused when the two upper chambers of the heart beat rapidly and unpredictably, producing irregular heartbeat.

A-Fib is a risk for stroke because it allows blood to pool in the heart. This tends to form clots which can be carried to the brain, causing a stroke.

Obstructive Sleep Apnea: Obstructive Sleep Apnea is more dangerous for men than women. This may be because more men suffer from the disorder and almost always at a younger age than women. Overall, sleep apnea doubles a man's risk of stroke. The risk increases with the severity of the disorder. Sleep Apnea is a sleep condition which includes loud snoring and breathing that stops and starts during sleep. The result is an interruption in breathing up to ten seconds and sometimes even more. This in turn decreases blood flow to the brain and can elevate blood pressure within the brain causing a possible hemorrhagic stroke. Obstructive Sleep Apnea can cause a whole host of health problems including A-Fib, high blood pressure, diabetes, etc., all of which are risk factors for stroke. Doctors and hospitals now have home testing devices for Obstructive Sleep Apnea.

Alcohol Abuse: Healthcare professionals can give no definite reason why drinking alcohol in excess may increase the risk of stroke, but scientists and healthcare professionals agree that drinking more than two drinks a day increases the risk of stroke. It is thought that alcohol contributes to thinning of the blood vessels and decreases efficiency of heart function which can cause a hemorrhagic stroke and clot formation.

Carotid Artery Disease: The carotid arteries are located in both sides of the neck. They supply blood to the brain, so when one side or both are clogged by a clot, an ischemic stroke will surely occur. Avoid other ischemic stroke risks such as obesity and smoking to lower risk of CAD. CAD is usually diagnosed by a doctor using a stethoscope to hear blood flow on either side of the neck.

Oral Contraceptives: Oral contraceptives nearly double the risk of stroke for women. Add obesity and smoking and the risk is much greater. I have mentored two women, one under forty, and one under thirty, who have had strokes that were attributed in part to oral contraceptives. How oral contraceptives can cause a stroke is not completely understood. Birth control pills now in use contain lower levels of estrogen than older versions. This has decreased the risk; however, risk factors should be discussed with the prescribing doctor.

Obesity and Belly Fat: Chapter 11 in this book is a near re-print of my September 2010 strokenetwork.org article. The studies that I quoted conclude that the correlation between increasing stroke incidence and increasing degree of obesity was apparent independent of other risk factors. Further, people with bigger waist circumference (belly fat) are at even greater risk.

Prior Stroke, TIA, or Heart Attack: All of these increase the risk for stroke so it is important to be under the care of both a primary care physician and a neurologist. A TIA or Transient Ischemic Attack is a mini stroke caused by the same risk factors as a stroke. A TIA usually lasts less than ten minutes but should be considered a warning for a stroke. Chapter 10 deals with TIA in more detail.

Lipoprotein A, Homocystenes, and C Reactive Proteins: There is increasing evidence that high levels of these are risk factors for stroke. When getting a simple blood test (CBC), doctors seldom include these three. Ask your doctor to include these for your next CBC.

<u>Arteriovenous Malformation and Cerebral Aneurism:</u> Malformation in the cerebral arteries, such as an AVM or an aneurism, can cause a vein to burst causing a hemorrhagic stroke.

The following sources were used in writing this chapter:

National Stroke Association:
www.stroke.org
American Heart Association:
www.americanheart.org
Science Daily:
www.sciencedaily.com
The National Institute of Health:
www.nih.gov
www.answers.com

Part II: Problems Associated with Stroke and TBI

Chapter 3: Strategies to Reduce Noise Sensitivity, Light Sensitivity, and Pain after Stroke

During the many years that I have mentored stroke and TBI survivors and attended many support group meetings, the problems of noise and light sensitivity, as well as pain after a stroke, have been talked about frequently. When I started researching this topic, I was introduced to a book titled <u>Learning to Live Again...One Day at a Time.</u> It is a book about the continued recovery of Chris Hotaling after he suffered a traumatic brain injury in 1999. The book was written by Chris along with his wife Amy and it is both inspirational and filled with ideas and suggestions for recovery. I recommend that everyone reading this chapter consider reading this book as well. It can be purchased at www.aspireplace.com.

While reading this book, I found a section that addressed the topic of this chapter and in turn I used this information extensively for this chapter. Chris and Amy offer simple and direct answers to the three problems listed above.

Light Sensitivity: Florescent lights, direct, bright sunlight, overcast skies, and sudden light from any source are all problems for some stroke and TBI survivors. Light can result in head and eye pain and the discomfort can last for a time after the light is eliminated. If this is a problem for you, Chris offers the following: Consider wearing sun glasses outside and also inside when the light is creating head and/or eye pain. Chris states, "If you enjoy reading and experience head or eye pain, you can find reasonably priced sunglasses that have a reading glass insert." If you have concerns with your vision, you should see a neuro-ophthalmologist to eliminate a diagnosis of a more serious eye disease.

Noise Sensitivity: Noise sensitivity is another frequent problem that stroke and TBI survivors face. Chris had major problems with this but was able to solve the problem. He learned that though foam earplugs can help, they can also muffle the sounds that you want to hear. His solution was molded ear filters. They do not block all of the noise, but instead reduce the highs, lows, and background noises allowing the users to enjoy conversations and concentrate on the sounds that they want to hear. Although there are many companies that offer ear filters, Chris obtained his from Sensaphonics (www.sensaphonics.com). Filters are available in different decibel ranges. See an audiologist to determine what is best for you.

Pain: This is a bit more difficult because pain can happen in a number of areas of the body, in varying degrees, and for various reasons. No doubt, if the pain is chronic, you have been to a doctor specializing in pain management. But if pain is persistent and you are looking for some general strategies, Chris offers the following:

Breathe: Seek out a quiet place, close your eyes, and eliminate distractions. Breathe in through your nose and exhale through your mouth. The goal is relaxation. You may want to refer to Chapter 15 about the benefits of yoga and meditation for people with disabilities.

Progressive Muscle Relaxation PMR: This is a step-by-step technique that helps you become aware of muscle tension and reduces the tension through a systematic approach that reduces pain. You may want to Google "PMR Exercise" which will bring you to web-sites that will show you visuals that walk you through the PMR exercises.

In January, 2013, I wrote an article for strokenetwork.org entitled "Chronic Headaches after a Stroke." I received an e-mail from a reader and stroke survivor who told me about a book entitled <u>The Trigger Point Therapy Workbook: Your Treatment Guide For Pain Relief</u> by Clair Davies. It was successful for this reader in eliminating pain after all else had failed. I looked up the book reviews from Amazon and almost every reader review gave it five stars. Also see Chapter 7, Dealing with headaches.

I must thank Chris and Amy Hotaling for providing the majority of the information for this chapter. Chris is presently a Personal Life Adjustment Coach and consultant for ASPIRE PLACE, a company he and his wife Amy founded. Chris and Amy give presentations and provide key-note-motivational speeches at conferences, workshops, and training programs throughout the United States. They can be reached by contacting Aspire Place at info@aspireplace.com.

Chapter 4: The Many Faces of Aphasia

Sandy had a stroke eleven years ago. She was left with paralysis in her right arm, weakness in her right leg requiring her to wear a brace to walk, and expressive aphasia. She understands what people are saying, but can only speak in short sentences, and usually expresses herself in one word. She cannot read, write, add, or subtract. These problems are common for people who have suffered a stroke or TBI on the left side of the brain which affects the right side of the body and communication abilities.

Cheinhwa had a stroke six years ago (he has since passed away from an unrelated illness), and had similar symptoms as Sandy. He also could understand when people spoke to him, but when he spoke, he struggled with every word. He could speak in complete sentences, but each sentence took a great deal of effort. He could read and write, but only slowly and with great effort.

Lucian had a TBI eight years ago. He was the victim of a violent assault. He was hit over the head with a blunt object (he is unable to remember what he was attacked with), and left for dead. He did recover but is cognitively impaired and has expressive aphasia. He also understands what people say, but he speaks so rapidly that it is difficult to understand him. He can read and write, but like Cheinhwa, he does so slowly and with some difficulty.

All of these survivors are people that I have mentored after being trained by the Brain Injury Alliance of New Jersey. They all have (or had in the case of Cheinhwa) aphasia but with different traits. And there are many other traits that I mention below giving aphasia "many faces." So what exactly is aphasia? If you research the term, aphasia is divided into many categories. The simplest way, however, is to divide aphasia into "expressive aphasia," which means the survivor has difficulty speaking, and "receptive aphasia," which means the survivor has difficulty understanding what is said. Some patients have symptoms of both.

Symptoms may include:

- Difficulty in pronouncing or forming words
- Difficulty understanding or comprehending language
- Difficulty or inability to read and/or write
- Tendency to repeat words or phrases
- Difficulty or inability to use complete sentences
- Difficulty or inability to repeat words or phrases
- Difficulty or inability to name or identify objects
- Poor enunciation

The most important point, however, is that any type of language problem as a result of a TBI or acquired brain injury is considered a form of aphasia.

If you have aphasia and are home after a hospital stay or in rehabilitation, what do you do? At some point speech therapists will decide there is little to gain from additional therapy sessions.

So now you must get on with your life. Here is what I recommend.

First, join a support group specifically for aphasia. Go to the National Aphasia Association website (www.aphasia.org) to find the support group nearest you. Scroll down under "aphasia community" to "aphasia community groups." Click on your state to get a list of support groups. Support groups are wonderful for sharing new techniques and meeting people with similar problems. If you cannot find a group close to you, start your own. The NAA web site tells you how.

Second, investigate the use of computer software and speech devices to see if they can help you continue with speech therapy on your own. Bungalow Software, Parrott Software, Communication Script Inc., and Lingraphica are examples.

Third, investigate clinics and community groups that specialize in aphasia. Again, on the NAA web site, scroll down under "aphasia community" to "aphasia programs and centers." This will enable you to see what is available in your state. Be sure you get details such as cost and success rate before you invest your money.

Hope for the Future

Pharmaceutical companies are testing drugs such as Piracetam, amphetamines, and Bromocriptine to improve speech for aphasia patients. Results are encouraging.

Neural Regeneration has also shown some promise. Researchers have used cell transplantation which is designed to restore brain tissue after a brain injury.

Constraint Induced Aphasia Therapy (sometimes called constraint induced language therapy) has also shown positive results. Many years after a stroke resulting in aphasia, studies have shown that CIAT has improved speech and comprehension in patients. During their therapy, the speech therapist spends three to four hours per day, five days per week, for three weeks giving intensive speech therapy targeting the patient's specific weaknesses.

I intentionally did not give details of these new advances because none of the studies are yet conclusive. However, if you want to find out more information on these and other studies, you can find it in an article entitled "Aphasia Therapy in the New Millennium" on the National Aphasia Association website.

Chapter 5: Falling: A Common Problem after Brain Injury

It first occurred to me that brain injury survivors face the risk of falling when I took a 42 year old stroke survivor to a restaurant in Philadelphia, Pennsylvania, for dinner. As we got up to leave, she slipped on the tile floor and took a terrible fall. Many people rushed over to help, but fortunately she was okay. I checked to see if the floor was wet. It was not. She had just lost her balance.

Another friend and stroke survivor is confined to a wheelchair, not because she cannot walk, but because she has chronic seizures and her doctor fears she will have a seizure and fall. Seizures are common in stroke survivors, and my friend told me she is in constant fear of falling.

I have since noticed that other brain injury survivors that have been affected by weakness in a leg often use a cane. Many times they never put the cane to the ground, but carry it as a sort of security blanket. This indicates a second problem. The fear of falling can interfere with the survivor's life style both physically and psychologically.

There have been many studies done concerning the danger of falling for stroke and TBI survivors. These studies show that between 36% and 40% of stroke survivors will fall depending on the study and the population that was used in that study. And as stated previously, the Center for Disease Control lists falls as the leading cause by far, of a TBI. These findings suggest that many stroke and TBI survivors will experience falls and perhaps multiple falls, and a significant number will sustain injuries. As a result, rehabilitation will be interfered with and the quality of life may be diminished.

Physical Therapist Jackie Harry, reported "...studies have shown that stroke survivors are twice as likely to fall following a stroke and more than three times as likely as the general population to fall multiple times." (Stroke Smart Magazine, Jackie Harry, Jan./ Feb.; pp. 6-7).

It is well documented that the reason for such a high incidence of falls among stroke and TBI survivors is twofold. One reason involves the impaired physical condition of the patient. The other is due to the living environment of the patient.

The physical condition is key. Weakness and loss of feeling on the affected side increases the possibility of falling. Other factors include proneness to dizziness, loss of vision, loss of balance, and overall poor health.

There are several things that can be done to decrease the risk of falling. Staying healthy by eating well, keeping slim, exercising, giving up smoking, and having regular eye exams are all important.

The patient's neurologist and primary care physician should also make fall prevention a part of routine care. And if a patient does fall, it is important not only to deal with the physical recovery, but also with the emotional recovery so he doesn't live in fear of falling again.

Dr. Edgar J. Kenton III, Director of the Stroke Prevention/Intervention Research Program at Morehouse University in Atlanta, Georgia, states, "The living environment of the patient, must also be examined, evaluated, and modified to lessen the chance of a fall." The environment may be the hospital, the nursing home, or the patient's private residence. If the patient lives at home, he or his caregivers must take responsibility for creating a safe home environment. Every room must be evaluated for safety.

The <u>Brain Injury Association</u> distributes a pamphlet called <u>Heads Up Seniors: A Guide to Preventing Falls.</u> It is a checklist to help seniors to prevent falls but it also applies to brain injury survivors.

Preventing Falls

- Keep the stairs, handrails, and stair coverings in good repair. and make sure walking areas, inside and out, are well lit.
- Remove throw rugs from your home or use double sided tape to secure edges to the floor.
- Remove ice, snow, and leaves promptly from walks and driveways and repair cracks in exterior walkway areas.

- Use anti skid mats in and around the tub or shower.
- Grab bars are a good idea near the toilet and in the shower.
- Reorganize items in work and storage areas to within easy reach.
- Remove obstacles from floors and walking areas. These include magazines, books, cords, and low furniture.
- Spills should be cleaned up immediately.
- Wear supportive, low heeled shoes.
- Review medications with your doctor or pharmacist for possible side effects and keep medicines well labeled.
- Exercise regularly, with your doctor's approval, to improve your strength and balance.

Chapter 6: Alexia: Learning to Read Again

Alexia is the term used when someone loses the ability to read or understand words, sentences, or in some cases, even letters. It is also called visual aphasia or word blindness. This is fairly common after a brain injury. It is caused by severe damage to the left side of the brain (the occipital and temporal lobes).

Alexia is a form of dyslexia but dyslexia is developmental, meaning that it does not happen from an occurrence such as a stroke or traumatic brain injury. Alexia is an acquired reading disability as a result of an acquired event such as a stroke. It is most common for alexia to be accompanied by expressive aphasia (the inability to speak in sentences), and agraphia (the inability to write).

All alexia is not the same, however. You may have difficulty with the following:

* Recognizing Words
* Difficulty identifying and reading synonyms
* Difficulty with reading despite your ability to sound out pronunciation of words
* Although you can read words, it is too difficult to read for very long
* Blind spots blocking the end of a line or a long word
* Focusing on the left side of the paragraph or page
* Double vision when trying to read
* Reading some words but not others. (Of course this makes reading impossible. I know a stroke survivor with alexia that can read larger words, but cannot read tiny words such as "it," "to," "and," etc.).

* Any combination of some of these traits

How do you combat alexia? Can it be fixed? Unfortunately, not much can be done about undoing alexia because there is not much scientific research that pinpoints the root cause. Further, even when a therapy works for one individual, it will probably not work for another individual. But there are things that you can do and try.

First, have a speech-language pathologist with experience with alexia do a formal diagnosis. He will be able to pinpoint the type of alexia that you have and suggest possible treatments and strategies. He will also be aware of the latest studies and treatments available.

Next, get a low vision examination by an ophthalmologist (not an optometrist) that has experience with alexia. If the problem is primarily damage to the visual field, he might be able to prescribe corrective lenses or be familiar with techniques to improve reading eye movements.

You can also try the following at-home treatments:*

Silent reading is easier than reading out loud. The difficulty of word retrieving in speech is also difficult for reading out loud.

Sound out individual letters and letter combinations. "s" would be the sssssss sound.

Combination sounds, which include "th" "sh" "ch" "st" "bl" "ph" "br" etc., require many practice sessions between the survivor and an aid.

Many words can be read correctly by sounding out the letters, then blending the sounds to make a word. In other words, learning to sound out the first letter can help in reading the entire word. Once you learn to sound out the first letter or combination, the letters can blend into words.

Some survivors are able to pronounce words that are spelled out to them. Start out with simple words such as c-a-r or h-a-t. Then move on to longer words such as a-n-i-m-a-l. Then move on to sentences such as l-o-o-k a-t- t-h-e a-n-i-m-a-l.

For nouns, try pairing the word with a picture of the object. The aid can then use these words in a sentence without the pictures so that reading takes place.

Some survivors cannot read due to visual attention. They cannot focus on one word at a time. Try cutting a window out of a piece of paper to block all but one word at a time.

Some patients can read words but they get confused as to when the line ends. By putting a solid book mark at the end of a paragraph, column, or page, these survivors may find that this method reduces confusion and helps in reading concentration. If the problem is finding the beginning of the sentence, put the book mark at the beginning of the paragraph, column, or page.

Other vision related alexia may be able to be corrected by the above ophthalmologist prescribing glasses.

If you read, but with difficulty, try large print books and magazines such as Reader's Digest Large Print. This helped a man that I know with alexia. You can also enjoy audio books which are readily available in book stores and libraries.

Note: I wish I could end this chapter by claiming that results of therapy are largely successful, but they are not. Studies are ongoing so perhaps there will be greater success in the future.

* Much of the information on at-home remedies came from the article, "Reading Rehab,"

by Margaret Greenwald, PhD, <u>Stoke Connection Magazine</u>, July/August, 2004.

Chapter 7: Dealing with Headaches

A woman writes to her doctor, "My husband had a left brain stroke four years ago. Rehabilitation has been a great success as he has regained 90% of the use of his limbs and almost all of his speech. However, he now suffers from chronic debilitating headaches. His only relief is to take the prescribed medication followed by a nap. Consequently, he spends much of his day in bed. Is this common after a stroke? Are these headaches a direct result of the stroke? Is this likely a permanent condition?"

Another woman writes, "I suffered a stroke last year and I am doing well except for chronic severe headaches a condition that I did not have prior to my stroke. I have been prescribed various medications and was even hospitalized where neurologists ran several more tests. The tests did not reveal any neurological problem and the doctors could not find a reason for my headaches." She asks, "Is there any remedy for this? Is this a common condition after a stroke?

I have read several other letters with similar complaints and the same questions, and have researched what various neurologists and headache specialists said in addressing this problem. I have also spoken to two neurologists to find out if there is a solution.

There was a wide difference in the answers that I received. One article that I read stated that about one third to one quarter of ischemic stroke survivors suffer from various degrees of headaches. Yet most of the other articles that I read and the two doctors that I talked to said that chronic headaches after a stroke are not common or even rare.

I found out that the headaches are usually bilateral affecting both sides of the head. Headaches are more likely when the stroke affects the cerebellum, the part of the brain that affects equilibrium and movement. In addition, patients who suffered from migraine headaches are more likely to suffer headaches after an ischemic stroke.

Dr. James Castle, a neurologist at NorthShore Health System in Chicago, stated "Headaches after a stroke are not very common, but they might occur for the following reasons:

- a redirection of blood flow when healthy arteries stretch and grow to supply blood to the part of the brain that has lost its normal supply
- stretching of the brain's covering from scarring, swelling, or atrophy of the brain
- small amounts of bleeding into the area of the old stroke (this is not likely)
- a small tear in an artery (this is rare)."

Dr. Castle also stated, "I have had several patients who get migraine headaches after stroke. The first thing I always try to do is make sure nothing dangerous is causing the headaches- usually this means getting an MRI of the brain and an MR angiogram of the blood vessels of the head and neck. Once it appears the headaches are benign, I treat them with preventative medications." (from, www.caring.com, October 1, 2011).

Dr. Uri Adler, a neurologist at Kessler Institute of Rehabilitation in New Jersey, said that chronic headaches after a stroke are not common. But if they exist, they are usually not permanent. He also recommended neurological tests be done to rule out a serious neurological problem and a vision evaluation to see if that is the underlying problem.

Dr. Marcia Dover, a neurologist in Hackettstown, New Jersey, agreed that chronic headaches after a stroke are not common at all. But if a patient suffers from headaches, and neurological problems have already been ruled out, then appropriate headache medications should be tried. She added that sometimes medications being taken for other conditions, especially if the patient is on multiple medications, can be the cause of the headaches.

In conclusion, I would say that if neurological and vision tests are negative, headache medications are the best chance for relief. There are so many different medications that it requires trial and error to find the right one. This can be narrowed down based on the type of headaches the patient gets: tension headaches, migraine headaches, or cluster headaches (the daily piercing pain that can last for days or weeks at a time.)

Chapter 8: Caregivers: Planning for the Future

I was at a fund raising dinner for ARC (the charity for those with developmental disabilities) with the county director, Bill Testa, when he mentioned that the average age of the population in group homes is in the 50's. The reason he gave was that parents are keeping their disabled children at home until they can no longer care for them or die.

I started to think: What happens to stroke and TBI survivors that cannot properly function on their own if their primary caregivers can no longer care for them or die? I interviewed over twenty caregivers of stroke and TBI survivors that were likely to die before their loved ones. All of them said that a nursing home or an assisted living home was not an option, or at least not a good option. When I asked them why, most said that it would devastate them to see their loved one in facility designed for and inhabited by the elderly. Also, in many cases, the cost would be paid for by Medicaid and facilities that accept Medicaid may not be the best.

Some of those that I interviewed said that they had no plan and would decide later. Others said that they expected that even though a facility was not a good option, it was probably what will happen. Still others said they hoped that a younger (or older) sibling would step in to the caregiver role. Some of this group had not secured approval from the sibling(s). And two that I interviewed said that the stroke or TBI survivor would probably not outlive them because of health reasons, and, therefore, had made no plans.

For example, I interviewed John*, a caregiver for his daughter Danielle, age 30. He told me that he and his wife considered this problem but are now at ease because his son and son's wife said they fully intend to care for Danielle if and when the time comes.

I interviewed Alan who told me that his son Steven's condition is severe and it is doubtful that he will outlive is parents. When I asked him what if he does, he said he hoped that his other children would do what is best for Steven, age 37.

Robert and his wife Gina told me that their son Ralph, age 47, will probably outlive them and will have to go into an assisted living home or a group home. They had not looked into anything as of yet.

Michael, caregiver and father of Greg, age 40, told me that this problem is constantly on his mind. His son cannot live on his own. His disability includes some cognitive impairment and obsessive compulsive disorder. An assisted living facility is out of the question because his son said he would never accept living with older people and would rather die. Yet there is no one who can be Greg's caregiver if Michael and his wife die.

What is important is that caregivers must plan ahead for this possibility. Assuming that your survivor is cognitively able to understand the subject, include him or her in the discussion. If siblings are a possibility, get ironclad approval that the survivor will be well taken care of by the sibling or siblings. If you decide that an assisted living facility is the option, visit places now and find out if there is a waiting list. There are also agencies that provide group homes for people with disabilities. The research and visitation should occur now, not later.

Caregivers must look at their options and plan now for the future. Get a plan, and follow up every couple of years. There may also be a support group for caregivers in your area. Attend a meeting and see what others have done about this problem. There are also many organizations on the internet to explore such as www.thefamilycaregiver.org. You can write for their advice on this and get a prompt response from other caregivers around the country. There is also a magazine called Today's Caregiver with helpful articles and columns.

*None of the names of caregivers and survivors are their real names.

Chapter 9: Aggressive Behavior after a Brain Injury

At some point after a debilitating stroke or TBI, the survivor may experience anger. It will vary as to the severity and the intensity, but anger of some degree usually happens.

But when anger is not controlled and when it becomes part of the survivor's personality, aggressive behavior can result. By aggressive behavior, I mean uncontrollable irritability, anger pointed at someone such as the caregiver, sudden outbursts without any reason, or, in some cases, unprovoked violence.

Jordan Grafman, PhD, has been researching the cause of this behavior in brain injured patients. He was on the staff of the Kessler Foundation Research Center until 2012. Dr. Grafman led a 2011 study published in the journal Neurology.

He and his team found that two main factors are the cause of aggressive behavior. The first is the location of the injury to the brain, and second, the behavior is influenced by genetics (predisposition) indicating that brain imaging and genetic testing can add to what we learn from psychological assessment.

Another study was led by Jong S. Kim, MD, Department of Neurology at Asan Medical Center in Seoul, South Korea. His findings agree with Dr. Grafman's. His study showed that aggressive behavior after a stroke is usually related to brain damage rather than from distress over their condition. In a study of 145 people who suffered a stroke, researchers found that those survivors that experienced anger or aggressive behavior (forty seven of the patients) had lesions on the parts of the brain responsible for producing serotonin, a brain chemical that moderates behavior. This study was also published in the journal Neurology.

Dr. Kim states, "To my mind, these anger symptoms are generally neurologic but not psychiatric, and doctors should explain this to patients and relatives who are disturbed by these behavioral changes."

Managing this aggressive behavior is important for recovery, the patients' relationships, and the patients' ability to work. It is also important for the caregivers' well-being. Dr. Grafman states, "Clinicians who see patients with lesions of the prefrontal cortex should inquire specifically about aggressive behavior." He adds, "Patients and their families may benefit from counseling or medication for the patient to manage this behavior. Short-term cognitive behavioral therapy can also be very helpful."

Caregivers may benefit from these tips:

+ Remember that aggressive behavior is part of the effects of the stroke. Your loved one cannot always control his behavior.
+ Stay calm. Do not overreact to your loved one's outbursts. Speak slowly and softly without raising your voice until your loved one calms down.
+ Avoid arguing with your loved one. Redirect his or her attention to something else.

+ After you find things that create anger in your loved one, avoid them as much as possible. For example, if you observe that being around a large amount of people sets him off, avoid that environment.
+ If you as a caregiver become angry or frustrated, back off and cool down. Chances are he or she will calm down after you step back and remain calm.
+ Stay safe. If your loved one becomes violent, back away. Keep a safe distance and seek help from a family member, a friend, or a neighbor if need be.

Many marriages break up after one spouse has a stroke or TBI. It is important that you have help with care giving. Don't wait for friends and family members to volunteer. Ask them to give you a break by caring for your loved one periodically.

Chapter 10: Risk of a Stroke after a TIA

Almost everyone who has had a stroke knows what a TIA is. A Transient Ischemic Attack, sometimes called a mini-stroke, occurs when a clot blocks blood flow and oxygen to the brain just as a stroke will do. The difference is in the length of time that the blockage is in place. In a TIA, the clot clears itself so that the stroke-like symptoms of the blockage are temporary.

Although the symptoms of TIA, such as numbness on one side of the face or body, blurred vision, slurred speech, dizziness, etc., usually last only for a short time, usually less than ten minutes, the TIA should be taken seriously. Studies have shown that patients are at risk of having a stroke after a TIA with the greatest risk coming within the first three days and, that between 24%

and 29% of patients who experience a TIA will have a stroke within five years if not treated.

Research suggests that between 500,000 and 600,000 strokes occur each year and approximately 10% of strokes are preceded by TIAs. Dr. S. Claiborne Johnston, Professor of Neurology at the University of California, San Francisco, stated at the 25th International Stroke Conference that "the acronym TIA should stand for Take Action Immediately." The symptoms of TIA often are not taken seriously by patients and physicians alike because they are usually short-lived and often mild. However, Dr. Johnston states, "TIAs are very, very, ominous." *

Betty Collins, a Registered Nurse and Facilitator of a support group at Kessler Institute in West Orange, New Jersey, concurs. Betty states, "I think many people just hope it goes away and when it does, they don't think about it again; even to the point of not mentioning it to their physicians." She adds that, "It is difficult for doctors to order a range of tests when symptoms are no longer present and a rationale for each test must be given."

I interviewed Dr. Sean Savitz, a neurologist at the University of Texas Medical Center in Houston, by telephone because I wanted to get first hand a doctor's perspective on TIAs. He emphasized that it is very important to seek medical treatment for a TIA to ascertain the patient's risk factors for a stroke such as high blood pressure, diabetes, etc. TIAs have different symptoms for different patients. Some TIAs result in drooping features on one side of the face, blurred vision in an eye, or tingling on one side of the body. Thus, people are not sure if they need treatment because they may not identify their particular symptoms as TIAs.

If you experience what you think might be a TIA, you should call for emergency medical service for immediate transport to a hospital equipped to care for people with stroke and TIA. Ideally, a PSC (Primary Stroke Center) is best. Never attempt to drive yourself to the hospital nor should you have a friend or relative drive you. If a medical complication occurs on the way to the hospital, EMS personnel are best trained to respond.

Diagnosis: Once the patient reaches the Primary Stroke Center or hospital, a complete neurological exam is called for.

This may include:

The standard Mini-Mental Status Exam to observe the patient's attentiveness, interaction with the examiner, language use, memory skills, etc.

A CT scan to identify any bleeding or mass that may be causing the symptoms.

An MRI (magnetic resonance imagery), to examine areas of the brain affected by the TIA.

An MRA (magnetic resonance angiogram) and/or an ultrasound to detect blockages or plaque build-up in the blood vessels. Special attention is paid to the carotid artery. If blockage is detected, removing plaque by surgery may be necessary.

A check for heart problems using an echocardiogram or an electrocardiogram (ECG).

Treatment: The treatment, of course, is determined after the results of the above mentioned tests are complete. Treatments vary from patient to patient. Since the goal is to prevent a stroke from occurring, great attention is paid to treat medical problems including high blood pressure, high cholesterol, smoking, and diabetes, which may have been the cause of the TIA in the first place. Other treatments include:

Anti-platelet therapy is a possible therapy to reduce the risk of platelet clumping and new clot formation. Dr.Nina Solinsky, of the University of Virginia Health Center states, "Aspirin is the most powerful anti-platelet drug available."

Other drugs may be added, such as dipyridamole (Persantine) if need be.

Anti-coagulant therapy is designed to decrease the risk of blood clots forming in the arteries. The most common of these medications is Warfarin (Coumadin). This type of medication is generally prescribed for patients who have had previous TIAs or are otherwise at high risk for a stroke.

Each year, about 240,000 people in the U.S. are diagnosed with a TIA. Recognize the symptoms so if it happens to you, you can take action.

Call 911 immediately. It may save your life or prevent a life of disability.

*This information comes from an article in FAMILY PRACTICE NEWS, April 15, 2000, by Eric Goldman.

Chapter 11: Obesity and Stroke

Part A: Obesity and Stroke Risk
This is a touchy subject. Most of us are overweight and some of us are obese. Do either of these conditions increase the risk of having a stroke? That is the question.

Dr. Hiroshi Yatsuya, a visiting professor at the University of Minnesota, Minneapolis, headed a study that examined this question. It followed 13,549 middle aged men and women in four United States communities from 1987 through 2005. The researchers used all three measures of obesity: body mass index, waist circumference (belly fat), and excess weight.

The conclusions were published in January, 2010 in <u>The Journal of the American Heart</u>

<u>Association</u>. Here are some of the major conclusions drawn by Dr. Yatsuya's team:

- The correlation between increasing stroke incidence and increasing degree of obesity was apparent regardless of race and gender.
- Since individuals with higher degrees of obesity tended to have higher blood pressure levels, diabetes prevalence, and higher cholesterol, which are all risk factors for stroke, it is difficult to conclude that obesity is a true factor causing stroke.
- The study results re-emphasize the need to prevent obesity in general. But, clinical trials would be needed to determine whether obesity prevention or control would actually decrease stroke incidence.

In another study * by a group of researchers from Brigham and Women's Hospital in Boston, it was determined that obesity is a direct risk factor for stroke. The conclusion of this study, headed by Dr. Tobias Kurth, and published in the <u>Harvard Gazette</u> in 2003, goes beyond Dr. Yatsuta's study, even though it took place earlier, because, as Dr. Kurth states, "….the stroke risk associated with weight gain has, until this study, been a debatable issue. We are now able to show that there is a quantifiable increase in your chances of having a stroke when you are overweight or obese." Furthermore, the study concluded that results were basically the same when an adjustment was made for other stroke risks such as high blood pressure, diabetes, and high cholesterol.

*this study included only men.

But either way, we all know how dangerous obesity is.

Obesity leads to:
- high blood pressure
- high cholesterol
- diabetes
- lack of exercise

All of which may increase the risk of a stroke.

Part B: Obesity and Recovery after Stroke
- If a survivor has weakness or spasticity in one leg, the obese patient is more likely to be in a wheelchair than a survivor that is not overweight or obese.

- Obese patients were less likely to be discharged directly home instead of to a rehab facility or nursing home.
- Obese patients are more likely to be in the hospital longer as they are recovering from a stroke than a patient who is not overweight.
- Balance, stamina, and mobility are more difficult for the survivor that is overweight or obese.

Part III: Living a Productive Life after a Brain Injury

Chapter 12: Joining a Support Group

From the first, this chapter is intended to convince the reader that attending a stroke or brain injury support group is a valuable experience. If you have already been to a support group meeting and did not like it, then I urge you to give it more than one try. If after you have gone to several meetings and still see no benefit, try a different group. If there is no support group near you, start one. More about how to do that later.

I have been a volunteer mentor to stroke survivors for the last twelve years. I started going to a support group seven years ago in an effort to introduce the experience of a support group to four survivors that I am mentoring. We all still go twice each month and have dinner together before the meeting. Even though I am neither a survivor nor a care-giver, I benefit by learning about problems, feelings, frustrations, new found abilities, and a host of other things that come up at each meeting. We all also love the social events organized by the facilitator and the group.

Probably the best way to convince you to seek a support group is for you to hear from survivors that I interviewed. I asked members of my support group in West Orange, New Jersey, and some from other support groups, what a support group means to them. Here are their answers.

"My support group is more like a family than just a group. It is a place that I can talk about problems that I do not want other people to hear. People in the group have the same or similar problems and I enjoy being with them." Matthew (Survivor)

"The support group makes me happy because they understand that I am lucky to be alive. The group helps me to understand that." Bill (Survivor)

"The support group means being with people who understand the challenges for a survivor and caregiver." Ellie (Bill's Wife)

"Since attending a support group, I have become enlightened. I hear of problems and many are similar to mine." Christopher (Survivor)

"A support group is a network of people with a common bond, which enables us to connect in the way a family does. A different sort of family, but an important one." Barbara (Survivor)

"Our support group is a network of people with a common bond. The group helps us to feel better and, like a family, we are there for one another." Arnold and Marie, (Barbara's Father and Stepmother)

"The support group is a very calming experience for me. I still remember the first time I walked into that (meeting) room and was met by Matt. I said to myself, 'OK I can do this.' I felt comfortable right away even though I was in total panic mode before. I have always felt closeness to the people there. Very few people understand like those in my group." Lisa (Survivor)

"My support group gives me a chance to exchange information about recovery therapies and the emotional and physical changes since my stroke. It also has meant making new friends with a common bond." Dave (Survivor)

"Stroke survivors share their stories and meet others who share their challenges. While I do not discount the counsel of medical and psychology professionals, there is no more effective counsel than that from another survivor in helping you move on with your life." David (Survivor)

"As a survivor, my support group is a place of true friendship and camaraderie. I have learned a lot from survivors with similar experiences following brain injury." Jane (Survivor)

"Through new friendships, we have shared many emotions experienced by all survivors and caregivers. As part of our participation, Jane and I have benefited from the input from others, and also believe our input has benefited others." Joe (Jane's Husband)

"With only a nod the group can understand the joy, the pain, the frustration, the hope, the worry, and the wonder of improvement and the sadness of disappointment with which we all live throughout the day." Ann and Al (Parents of Len; Len is a Survivor)

"When we saw other people in the group speaking about their problems, we felt ours were manageable. It is great to have others you can turn to. No problem is too small or too big to solve." Rita and Dan (Rita is a Survivor)

<u>Finding a Support Group:</u>

There are far fewer stroke support groups than there are brain injury support groups. Brain injury support groups generally have many stroke survivors in the group and can be just as beneficial as a stroke support group.

To find a stroke support group in your area:

http://www.strokeassociation.org

Click on "Life after Stroke" (Red Bar)

Scroll down to "Find a Support Group in Your Area"

To find a brain injury support group in your area:

Go to your state brain injury association.

For example, North Carolina's is
http://www.bianc.net.

Each state organization will have a place to click on to "find a support group."

Starting a Support Group: If you cannot find a support group that is close enough, consider starting one. There are two sources that I recommend.

First, there is an on-line 30 page booklet which is excellent. Go to: http://www.strokeassociation.org; Click on "Life After Stroke;" Click on "For Support Group Leaders" ---"Starting a Support Group;" Click on "Successful Support Groups" This brings you to the 30 page booklet.

Second, Deb Therault wrote a three part article entitled "Support Groups 101 for the strokenetwork.org in the following issues:

Part I, Determine Your Goal, Nov 2009

Part II, Setting the Stage, Dec 2009

Part III, <u>Making it Happen</u>, Jan 2010

I hope my survivor support group friends that contributed to this article have convinced you that a support group will be a positive experience in your life.

Chapter 13: The Benefits of Having a Mentor

Caregivers simply cannot do it alone.

If you are a stroke or TBI survivor, you were probably first stabilized in a hospital. Then you went to a rehabilitation center. After you had advanced to a certain point, or your insurance ran out, you went home. Whatever your disability, you began the process of adjusting to your new life. You had probably been an active person. You may have worked, volunteered, or traveled. In short, you probably were a busy person.

I have been a mentor to several stroke and traumatic brain injury survivors for eleven years. Over the years I have learned that two issues need to be addressed. First, survivors have difficulty coping with so much idle time. And second, the survivor wants to gain as much independence as possible.

Each survivor has different problems, disabilities, and needs. I cannot define exactly what a mentor does, but I can tell you what I think a mentor can do. First, the mentor becomes a friend to the survivor. That is why it is usually best if the mentor is of the same sex and about the same age. This isn't absolutely necessary as I have had success with females and with survivors both older and younger than me.

Second, the mentor should help the survivor establish goals to be achieved during the next six months or the next year. I discuss goals later in this chapter.

Third, a mentor should be able and willing to spend time with the survivor. This is sometimes difficult because the potential mentor may work and surely has family obligations. Ideally, however, a mentor should talk weekly on the phone to the survivor and take the mentor out for coffee or lunch at least twice per month.

Fourth, a mentor is someone who is there to listen to your problems and to help you to make decisions that will enhance your life.

My early contact as a mentor with a stroke or TBI survivor includes weekly telephone calls, weekly e-mails, letters that include articles on stroke, holiday cards, and occasional meetings for lunch or at a support group. Later, I help them with three objectives.

1. Establish daily and weekly routines: Get up in the morning the same time every day. This prevents the tendency to stay in bed too long, which can lead to boredom and depression.
2. Concentrate on Independence. Do as much for yourself as possible. This has both mental and physical benefits.
3. Establish goals. Goals might include:

   Find and use a county or local bus service, if you do not drive, so you can get around on your own.

   Join a support group and attend monthly meetings.

Take a course for fun at the local adult school, high school, technical school, or community college.

Try art as therapy. Get a color by numbers kit from your local department store. If you enjoy that, progress to a basic art class often offered at an art studio or a continuing education facility.

Exercise at a gym. See if the local hospital or "Y" has a program. Go two or three time a week as your regular routine.

Get a part-time job. Each state has a department specifically for people with disabilities to help you find a job.

Do some volunteer work. Go to volunteer-match.com, a nationwide web site that will point you to volunteer needs in your geographic area.

Of course the above goals are just some examples. You must establish your own goals to meet your needs and interests.

I describe below how I mentor three different survivors with different needs and disabilities.

Sandy: Sandy had an Ischemic (clot) stroke eleven years ago leaving her with a paralyzed right arm, an affected right leg making it necessary for her to walk slowly with a brace, and expressive aphasia making it difficult for her to talk and read. She does not have a caregiver and most of her family lives too far to help. I take her out to lunch each week. I take her to support group meeting twice per month (goal). I help her with bills and make sure she has her meds each month. I was able to help her get housing assistance (goal). I got her to join a gym for exercise (goal). I spend more time with Sandy than any of my other survivors because she has little other help and she lives close to me.

Chris: Chris also had an ischemic stroke four years ago. Together, we established four goals. First, I was able to help him regain his driver's license. This required that he get an evaluation followed by driving lessons at the Kessler Institute for Rehabilitation Driving School. Second, I helped get him his own apartment so he could live independently. Third, he started working a part-time job which helped with the fourth goal, buying his own car. I talk to him on the phone frequently and see him at least once each week.

Lucian: Lucian was the victim of a crime. He was hit over the head with a blunt object putting him in a coma for several months. He has some memory loss and has expressive aphasia. He also has some other cognitive deficiencies. When I became his mentor several years ago, I saw his biggest problem was idle time. So we set up goals together with his caregiver Patty. Now he is in a camera club and participates in a creative expo every June (goal). He rides horses at a handicapped riding center (goal). He belongs to a gym (goal). And he lives in an apartment with help from Patty (goal). Patty, Lucian and I have lunch or dinner together about twice each month.

All mentors cannot put in the time necessary to do all that they would like. But whatever they can do is beneficial. Two things can and should be accomplished: the survivor's life should be better. The caregiver gets a break by getting free time.

How can you get a mentor? Finding the right mentor takes perseverance. Here are some suggestions. Access your state brain injury association to see if they have a mentoring program. If they do, check to see what they allow the mentor to do. Ask the priest, minister, or rabbi to place an announcement in their bulletin. Put a notice on various bulletin boards in the various local hospitals, especially rehabilitation hospitals. If you join a support group, ask the members and the facilitator for advice on finding a mentor. Perhaps you can share this chapter with the group. College students are always ready to volunteer. If you think a young person would be appropriate, most colleges have a student wide system where a message can be sent to every student at once. In all of your efforts to find a mentor, include your e-mail address so if someone responds, you can e-mail them back with this chapter so they will understand what a mentor should do. My last suggestion is to find another stroke survivor at your support group and see if they might be interested in a weekly lunch date and periodic get together to attend social events.

Chapter 14: Therapeutic Horseback Riding

If you are a stroke or TBI survivor or someone who cares for a stroke or TBI survivor, I fear you might skip this chapter because you cannot imagine someone who has had a stroke or TBI being able to ride a horse. You may think that your disability would make riding a horse impossible. You may think you are too disabled or too old, or that you have never ridden a horse. But for those who have taken part, the rewards are invaluable.

Survivors all over the U.S. and Canada are enjoying the fun, the thrill, and the therapeutic benefits of riding on a horse at one of the hundreds of therapeutic riding centers designed exclusively for people with disabilities. Try finding a center accredited by the Professional Association of Therapeutic Horsemanship (PATH), formerly the North American Riding for the Handicapped

Association (NARHA). They list the locations of handicapped riding centers and you can find the location nearest you on the web at www.pathintl.org.

"Try it once and you are hooked," says Lucian, a TBI survivor who has both cognitive and physical disabilities. He rides at Freedom Horse, a center in Long Valley, New Jersey. Elizabeth Carlson is the owner of Freedom Horse and she explains the therapeutic value of riding for a survivor like Lucian. "Riding a horse is like adding an extension to your own body."

Lucian, whose disability is mostly cognitive, with some limb weakness, is able to control both sides of the horse. This allows him to ask his horse (Murphy) to move at his pace. He tells him where he wants to go without worrying about the disability not taking him there. Therapeutic Riding does not focus on what you cannot do; it focuses on how you can do it. That's the value, being able to do something you thought you would never be able to do.

But let's not lose sight of the fun of riding. Yes, it has therapeutic physical value as already stated.

However, it has emotional value by helping the rider overcome fear and anxiety and increase his self esteem. It has cognitive value as the rider learns to give commands to the horse. Speech and language skills can be practiced in this fun and challenging environment. Every rider I have interviewed, talks about how much fun it is to ride.

Available Programs

Although all facilities across the US and Canada do not offer all of the programs listed below, they all offer one or more. You should check with the facility nearest you to see what programs it offers.

Therapeutic Riding

Individuals with almost any cognitive, physical, or emotional disability can benefit from therapeutic riding. It is supervised, recreational horseback riding designed to improve balance, coordination, stamina, and confidence. The emotional and psychological benefits are primarily the result of meeting the challenges presented by riding and achieving goals while striving to accomplish riding independently. Riding also has the benefit of human/animal bonding. This bonding is evident with Lucian and Murphy.

Therapeutic Vaulting

Therapeutic Vaulting is an activity whereby a group of individuals engage in a variety of gymnastic positions on the back of a horse, as well as performing movements around, on, and off the horse. The horse is specially trained and each class is typically led by a licensed therapist and a riding instructor. According to Beverly Willard, a physical therapist at the Maryland Therapeutic Riding Center, benefits of therapeutic vaulting include aerobic conditioning, motor development, body awareness and coordination, increased confidence, and teamwork skills.

This method surpasses the therapeutic riding of a horse by teaching the basic vaulting positions along with exercises determined by the needs of the individual. Participants usually work in a group but each rider can progress at his own pace.

Hippotherapy

Hippotherapy is a treatment that uses the multi-dimensional movement of the horse to administer physical or occupational therapy. In hippotherapy the horse influences the rider rather than the rider controlling the horse. The goal is to get the rider to respond to the horse's movement or gait. The therapist uses this treatment to improve the rider's posture, coordination, strength, balance and equilibrium.

Specifically, hippotherapy will strengthen the muscle groups used every day in walking, sitting, and reaching. The therapist may have the rider stand up on the stirrups, lean forward, lean backward, throw a ball at a target, and any number of additional activities all while riding the horse. Parents of children engaging in hippotherapy notice improved confidence and overall happiness. Specific riding skills are not taught as in therapeutic riding, but rather a foundation is established to improve neurological function and sensory processing.

Carriage Driving

Carriage Driving is available in some facilities for people with disabilities which would not allow them to ride. It offers an alternative means of enjoying the company of a horse. The disabled driver is accompanied by an able-bodied "whip" in an open carriage. The experience offers the disabled driver the feeling that he is in control as he has a set of reins along with the "whip."

Find More Information: Check out these websites:

US Driving for the Disabled (USDFD)
   www.usdfd.org

Professional Association of Therapeutic Horsemanship (PATH); www.pathintl.org

Find a Center: www.pathintl.org; click "find a center."

Chapter 15: Yoga for People with Disabilities

I started writing an article on fitness after a stroke and discovered there is a wealth of information out there giving great advice on keeping fit with exercise. I had almost completed the article when a member of my support group introduced me to adaptive yoga for people with disabilities. I began reading about this and realized that it would be better if I could see an adaptive yoga class in action.

The class was instructed by Della Moses Walker who was trained specifically to teach adaptive yoga at the Wellness and Enrichment Center in West Orange, New Jersey.

Many of the participants were stroke or TBI survivors. The emphasis was on the individual. The pace for progress was slow so that each individual could advance at his own pace.

Della emphasized the following:

Yoga is a mind body connection.

Yoga with meditation yields relaxation of the mind and body.

Breathing in yoga is an important element for relaxation and concentration.

Adaptive yoga is designed to fit individual ability.

Two common problems for stroke and TBI survivors are balance and weakness affecting an arm, a leg, or both. The yoga instructor, Della, circulated and gave instruction to each participant as needed. Some students were able to sit on the floor as a regular yoga class would begin. Others were able to lie on a mat. Some were able to stand holding on to the back of a chair, while others sat in chairs.

In yoga, there are many yoga poses (specific positions) that the instructor uses. The goal is to improve balance, strength, flexibility, mobility, and to create an environment of relaxation through breathing techniques. Following are examples of exercises for chair yoga taken from Shirley Marotta, www.livingwordsofwisdom.com.

Chair Yoga

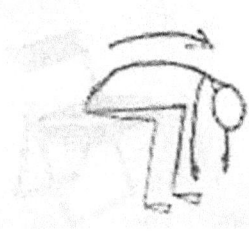

Forward Bend – eases tension in the upper back and neck. Breathe in and out as you bend forward. Let your head and arms hang over your knees. Relax into the position and hold for a few seconds and keep breathing. Breathe in as you slowly come back to a seated position.

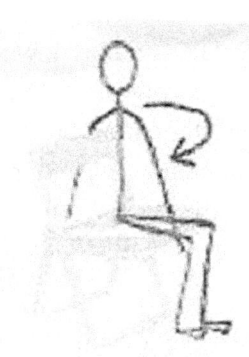

Spiral Twist – increases circulation and flexibility in the spine. Sit facing forward placing your left hand on the outside of your right knee. Place the opposite arm over the back of the chair. Breathe in and breathe out as you twist your body to the right

Turn your head as well. Push against your knee with your hand. Breathe normally and hold that position. Release slowly and come back to facing forward. Repeat on the opposite side if you are able.

Chair Yoga

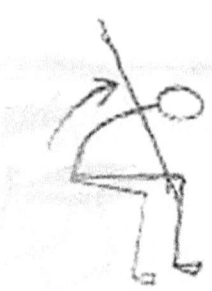

Side Stretch – increases flexibility of the spinal column, improves respiration, and reduces waistline. Sit facing forward with feet slightly apart, breathe in, and raise your arms out to both sides.

Breathe out and bend to the left, reaching toward the floor with your left hand and your right hand pointing toward the ceiling. Breathe in and come back to the starting position. Repeat with the right side.

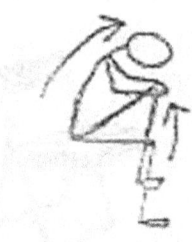

Knee Squeeze – relaxes lower back, improves digestion and respiration. Breathe out and breathe in and put both hands around the front of your knee. Pull your left knee to your chest while holding in your breath.

Lower your head to your knee and hold for a few seconds. Then release slowly while breathing out. Repeat on your right side.

Chair Yoga

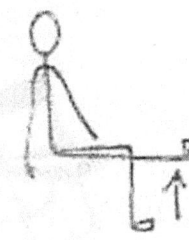

Leg Lifts – strengthens legs and lower back, and improves circulation to your legs and feet. Sit and hold each side of the chair for balance. Breathe out and breathe in as you lift straightened left leg and flex your foot. Hold for a few seconds and then slowly breathe out while lowering your leg. Repeat with your right leg.

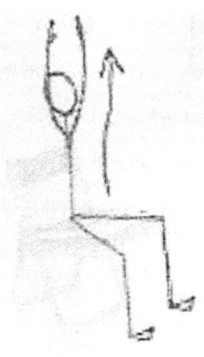

Sun Pose – improves circulation to your head, massages internal organs, and limbers your spine and hips. Sit back in the chair with legs apart and arms by your side.

Breathe out completely then breathe in and with a sweeping motion bring your arms up over your head. Look up and stretch. Breathe out while bending forward between your legs and if possible, put your palms on the floor.

Slowly breathe in while rising back up with your arms over your head again, then lower your arms to the side.

Although the above chair exercises are beneficial, they are no substitute for adaptive yoga classes because the instructor will pattern your exercises to meet your individual abilities and needs. You can find out where you can participate in adaptive yoga classes through the closest rehabilitation hospital. You may also see if anyone in the local support group knows of such a program.

There are also two sources you may want to consider. The first is a video called, <u>Yoga: Renewal of Life</u>, by the Rocky Mountain Stroke Center. Second is a book, <u>Recovery Yoga: A Practical Guide For Chronically Ill, Injured, and Post Operative People</u> by Sam Dworkis.

Chapter 16: Fitness after a Brain Injury

The previous chapter was about yoga for people with *disabilities. This chapter discusses other ways to keep fit after a stroke or TBI.*

While mentoring several stroke and TBI survivors over the past ten years, it occurred to me that anyone who has suffered a physical disability as a result of a stroke or TBI may experience spasticity of one or both legs, or of one or both arms, and cannot get the exercise that they should. I have written this chapter for stroke and TBI survivors who seek ways to exercise despite their disability.

You can organize an exercise program at home, a local gym or the local "Y." The important thing is that you work out consistently, safely, and in a way that addresses your physical needs. Although you may not want to address all of the points in this chapter, you should review each point to determine your needs.

If you decide to work out at home, be sure that you are exercising safely. I recommend that you speak to a fitness specialist or Physical Therapist to be sure that you are exercising correctly. If you join a facility, (a gym or the "Y"), be sure the fitness staff member knows something about stroke and TBI rehabilitation. Perhaps you can ask for someone who might be most suitable.

When developing a program that addresses the needs of most survivors with spasticity, include strength training, balance, flexibility, posture, and cardiac conditioning.

Strength Training: This area requires equipment such as weight machines, dumbbells, free weights, a padded gripping device, a squat machine, and a weight and pulley machine. You may want to start with just dumbbells because they are easy to use, they are safe, and you can do multiple upper body exercises with them. Be sure to increase weight gradually.

Balance: Every stroke and TBI survivor that I have mentored has some problem with balance. There are many exercises to address this problem. I recommend that you consult a fitness expert to get the best exercises for you. The advantage here is that most or all of these exercises can easily be done at home. I have worked with two stroke survivors with balance issues and found two effective exercises: stepping up and down on an adjustable step, and walking in a line heel to toe for about 20 feet. It is important, however, that you always have a spotter when working on balance.

Flexibility: Flexibility requires stretching. To stretch affected muscles and joints you will need a partner to help you. Your regular daily activities do not include flexibility stretching so this part of your program is important.

Posture: I am reluctant to include this element as part of your exercise program, but I did so because muscle, balance, and vision changes from your stroke or TBI can lead to poor posture. When walking with a cane, there is a tendency to look down. Try to look up as much as possible while exercising. When walking, concentrate on good posture.

Cardiac Conditioning: All exercises have some cardiac benefit. However, if you have access to a treadmill, it is a great cardiac conditioner with the added benefit of balance training. Of course, having a spotter is essential. A stationary bike is a close second to the treadmill for cardiac work.

Although few studies have been done concerning the benefit of exercise for stroke survivors. I cannot imagine a doctor not recommending an exercise program barring some other condition present which would make it dangerous to exercise.

Chapter 17: The Feldenkrais Method

The Feldenkrais Method was developed by Moshe Feldenkrais, a Russian physicist; who in 1919 immigrated to Palestine. He later lived in Paris, the UK, and finally in Tel Aviv, Israel. He began developing his "Method" in the 1940's which he then characterized as "Mind and Body." By the 1950's he began teaching his "Method" which we now know as The Feldenkrais Method.

The Feldenkrais Method is designed for anyone who wants to improve movement, flexibility, and physical function. Its purpose is to help reduce pain and limitations in movement. Lessons usually take place in a group led by a trained practitioner and last between 30 and 60 minutes. These group lessons are called "Awareness Through Movement." There are hundreds of lessons, usually conducted while sitting in a chair or lying on the floor. The "Awareness Through Movement" lessons differ from massage and chiropractics. Where massage concentrates on muscles and chiropractics adjusts the bones, the Feldenkrais Method works with movement through the nervous system.

Using the group method "Awareness Through Movement," lessons involve thinking, moving, and imagining. Each lesson consists of gentle, easy movements that gradually increase range and complexity. "Awareness Through Movement" lessons vary in difficulty from simple to demanding depending on how much the participant can handle.

It is worth the effort to watch some video demonstrations. There are many available. My favorites are:

Google **Grace and Feldenkrais**
Google **Mary Spire Feldenkrais Method**. On the left hand side (purple), click on "U-Tube Videos." There is a video demonstrating "Awareness Through Movement," and a video demonstrating individual lessons called "Functional Integration."

I found out about the Feldenkrais Method from Carrie Freed who gave a fifteen minute demonstration to our Support Group. Carrie is an occupational therapist and a certified Feldenkrais practitioner. The demonstration centered on the neck and shoulders. When finished, I had greatly improved range of motion in my neck. That was after just fifteen minutes. I Interviewed Carrie to get insight on how the Feldenkrais Method has helped stroke and TBI survivors.

Q: Stroke and TBI survivors have many different physical handicaps. What type of physical disability responds best to the Feldenkrais Method?

A: With time and patience I have found all disabilities can respond to the Feldenkrais Method (FM). The lessons taught in both "Awareness Through Movement" and "Functional Integration" help develop better awareness of oneself from a physical, sensory, and cognitive perspective. All change takes time. In my experience, it is the small changes over time that adds up to big changes in the months and years ahead.

Q: How much success have you had working with stroke and TBI survivors using the Feldenkrais Method?

A: Success post-stroke or TBI is defined differently for everyone who has experienced a stroke or TBI. In the area of strokes or TBI, I like to think of success as CHANGE. If a person is not satisfied with how he is functioning, then being static is "bad" and CHANGE is "good." The changes can be subtle ("I have a better sense of where my leg is today") and over time, that can be built upon ("I can place my leg a little better when I'm walking so I feel more steady.")

Q: For stroke or TBI survivors, should the Feldenkrais Method be combined with physical therapy and/or occupational therapy?

A: Physical Therapy and Occupational therapy use a medical approach to stroke rehabilitation. FM focuses on experiential (experience) learning combined with research, science and medicine. The stroke or TBI survivor may receive different ideas from the PTs and OTs than from the Feldenkrais practitioners. The combination of knowledge is valuable, especially since the recovery after a stroke or TBI is not a straight line or a recipe. What works for one person may not work for another.

Q: For stroke and TBI survivors, does the Feldenkrais Method work better shortly after the brain injury or can it be effective some time later?

A: Our brains are changing all the time. It's called brain plasticity. The idea that almost all recovery happens within the first year after stroke is an old idea. What does happen is that "habits" form. How we sit, how we walk, how we form our words, are strongly engrained in our nervous system and brain. As functions of the brain move away from the damaged area of the brain, FM is used to break these habits that were formed early on after the stroke or TBI.

Another source of information came from Barbara Natali, a member of my support group. She was a participant in a group taught by Carrie Freed. Barbara told me that she practiced "Functional Integration" (one on one) with Carrie for about two years. She believes the Feldenkrais method resulted in great improvement in mobility. Barbara stated, "Prior to Feldenkrais, I was unable to roll over in my bed. Through my work with Carrie, I was able to roll over and get out of bed." When I met Barbara several years ago, she was in a wheel chair. She now walks without even the use of a cane. She credits the Feldenkrais Method combined with intense physical therapy for this improvement.

Although the Feldenkrais Method was designed for those who want to improve the ability to move parts of their body freely, stroke and TBI survivors who have lost flexibility or suffer pain or discomfort when walking, turning, lifting, or just moving about, should give the Feldenkrais Method a try.

Chapter 18: Telerehabilitation

Telerehabilitation should not be confused with telephone intervention, both of which are being implemented with stroke and TBI survivors. Typically, telephone intervention is designed to help caregivers who need help in solving problems related to their role. This takes place after a home visit by a trained nurse shortly after the patient is discharged from an in-patient facility, and is followed by periodic (usually weekly) telephone contacts.

This chapter, however, centers on actual rehabilitation using the telephone, e-mail, or other electronic communication devices. It is based on the studies of three researchers:

Dr. Tim Johansson, Paracelsus Medical University, Salzburg, Austria;

Gitendra Uswatte. Professor of Psychology at the University of Alabama Birmingham, and principal investigator for the Telerehabilitation grant from the NIH (National Institute of Health)

Dr. Edward Taub, University Professor of Psychology in the Department of Psychology, and Director of the Taub Clinic at the University of Alabama Birmingham

Telerehabilitation is a method that provides rehabilitation services to patients who cannot easily receive it at a rehabilitation hospital due to distance, lack of trained physicians nearby, or patient mobility difficulties. Studies are presently being done with real patients to provide rehab to stroke survivors when one arm and/or hand has been affected. Through Telerehabilitation, Constraint Induced Movement Therapy (CIMT) has been used successfully to improve the use of the affected limb. CIMT is a method by which the patient is encouraged to increase use of the affected arm by asking him to wear a large mitt on the unaffected hand in the treatment setting and at home, and rewarding use of the affected arm in both settings. When a stroke or TBI occurs that weakens one arm, normal tasks using that hand and arm are lost. Later, that ability returns, but the brain has learned that it cannot control that limb. Dr. Edward Taub calls this "learned disuse. "The goal of CIMT is to retrain the brain to use the affected limb. *

The problem with CIMT is that it requires many hours of one-on-one therapy with a trained therapist. That is often impossible for many stroke survivors. So Dr. Taub, with Dr. Peter Lum and colleagues, has created a device that automates the delivery of CIMT called AutoCITE. The second generation of this device, which Dr. Uswatte, Dr. David Brennan, and colleagues also made contributions to, looks like a small computer desk with a monitor, three webcams, and a board with knobs and buttons used for practicing eleven different upper extremity tasks. Preliminary studies show that using AutoCITE is as effective as standard CIMT and reduces the time and effort of the therapist by 75%. This suggests that a trained therapist would be able to work with several patients at once. *

I communicated via e-mail with Dr. Johansson and Dr. Uswatte and asked each of them three questions.

Q. Is Telerehabilitation being used on a wide scale?

A. Both Doctors said that Telerehabilitation is being used in the form of studies. It is not being used as therapy yet.

Q. Do you need special equipment in the home to implement Telerehabilitation?

A. Dr. Uswatte and his team are using AutoCITE. Dr. Johansson added that the hope for the future is to have the device in community centers, hospitals, and clinics close to the patient's home.

Q. Is Telerehabilitation designed for upper and lower extremity improvement?

A. Both Doctors said that the studies that are on-going are focusing on upper extremities only.

Several studies are on-going, and preliminary results are encouraging. An on-going Telerehabilitation trial of CIMT using AutoCITE suggests this approach is a feasible method for providing arm rehabilitation in the home. A case study from this trial has been presented at a conference.

+ the subject was nine years post stroke

+ the subject received intense therapy (CIMT) for three hours each day for eight days.

+ restraint of the non-effected arm (using a mitt) was in place for 90% of waking hours.

+ tasks were made more difficult starting in day seven.

+ the subject consistently improved arm movement and use culminating after the eighth day.

You can see this case study and other studies on the internet by Googling "Edward Taub" or "Constraint Induced Movement Therapy."

Dr. Johansson concludes, "The over-all quality of research on outcome measures has been used. In order to compare the result of the studies, a harmonization of study design is recommended. More research involving a greater number of participants is required to determine effectiveness and costs and the utilization of telerehabilitation services in post stroke care."

You can learn more about Dr. Johansson's research by viewing his article, "Telerehabilitation in Stroke Care – A Systematic Review," Journal of Telemedicine and Telecare, 2011; 17: 1-6.

If you or someone you know has had a stroke that affects an upper extremity limb, you may be interested in the progress of Telerehabilitation studies. Perhaps Telerehabilitation using Constraint Induced Movement Therapy will be available in the near future in your home or at a clinic near you.

* These two paragraphs were taken primarily from an article published in the Birmingham (Alabama) News on September 8, 2011, by Hannah Wolfson.

Chapter 19: SIRROWS

SIRROWS or Stroke Inpatient Rehabilitation Reinforcement of Walking Speed is a recently completed study that addresses whether coaching stroke patients with weakness in one leg can increase walking speed and, therefore, improve quality of life. This was the first international trial to test a simple intervention for stroke rehabilitation. The group hopes to carry on others. The study did not require any funding.

July, 2009. The study was headed by Dr. Bruce Dobkin, Director of Neurologic Rehabilitation at the UCLA Medical Center in Los Angeles, California. The study consisted of two groups totaling 184 patients in eighteen study locations throughout the world. Of the 184 participants, 87% had had ischemic strokes. The distribution of left brain strokes versus right brain strokes was about even.

One group, called the "DRS Group," (Daily Reinforcement of Speed) received the customary therapy and daily reinforcement by their physical therapist. These patients were timed with stopwatches each day (usually several times during the session) while walking for a distance up to 25 feet. The patients were encouraged to walk faster each day and after each attempt, the therapists provided encouragement by such comments as "you improved by x seconds today," or "you are walking better every day."

The second group, called the "NRS," (No Reinforcement of Speed), received customary therapy and walked up to 25 feet but was not timed and received no reinforcement about walking speed. A comparison was made at the conclusion of the study after all data was collected.

Results of the Study
Patients in the DRS group improved their walking speed significantly when compared to the "NRS" group, at the time of discharge and even more so after three months post discharge.

Many from the DRS group achieved community level walking speeds by the time of discharge.

Since this type of rehabilitation does not require funding or special training for implementation, individual rehabilitation facilities could begin their own studies or implement a SIRROWS type program while a subject is an inpatient. Subsequent studies are being conducted on a large scale and SIRROWS is being used more frequently in facilities around the world.

There are still at least two unanswered questions however. Will the patients continue to improve or at least maintain their level of improvement after the three month measured study results? And, can patients that are several years post stroke also benefit from daily reinforcement of speed?

If you would like to see the details of this study, go to the following:

www.clinicaltrials.gov; click on "Search For Clinical Trials;
type in "SIRROWS."

SIRROWS also has a newsletter on-line designed to keep you informed as to progress of the studies and results of the therapy.

I want to extend a special thank you to Dr. Daniel Kalemba, PT, DPT, Kessler Institute of Rehabilitation, West Orange, New Jersey, and Dr. Bruce Dobkin MD, UCLA Geffen School of Medicine for their help in writing this chapter.

Chapter 20: Friends: Where Did They All Go

"After my stroke, many friends came to visit me in the hospital and in the re-hab facility. But after a while, my friends were not around anymore. When my wife called them, they always had an excuse."

"I had plenty of support in the hospital, but once I came home, the contact stopped. I haven't seen any of them for years."

"I lost most of my friends, maybe because I have aphasia and speaking is difficult. The few friends that I still have don't understand my difficulties and they don't try to communicate with me."

These are not direct quotes from any one person. They are typical, however, of some of the comments that I hear from stroke and TBI survivors.

For the last twelve years I have been mentoring Sandy Smethers, a 52 year old single mother of two. She had her stroke twelve years ago and, at the time, I did not know her very well. The stroke left her right arm paralyzed and weak in her right leg. She is able to walk without help, but at a slow pace. She also has expressive aphasia which makes speaking very difficult.

When I first went to see her in the hospital in December, 2000, she had many visitors who introduced themselves as friends of Sandy. Later, when she came home, these friends and more, told me they intended to stick with her as life-long friends. As time went on, however, most of these friends disappeared. So I asked myself, "Where did they all go?"

Why do friends disappear in so many cases?

Keeping friends depends on many variables.

- How many friends did you have before the stroke or TBI?
- Are you living with your wife/husband, your family, or do you live alone?

- What are your disabilities as a result of your stroke or TBI?

I asked several survivors, caregivers, and professionals about why they thought friends disappear after a stroke. Here is what they said.

- Some friends are uncomfortable seeing a once strong person that is now suffering with a disability which is sometimes extreme. It might be similar to visiting a cancer patient that has little time to live. It is easier to avoid the discomfort.
- A stroke alters a person's life. It can change the survivor's values, goals, attitudes, etc. When these changes occur, whatever the survivor and friend had in common in the first place, may be lost after the stroke.
- Sometimes, different emotions that are the result of the stroke or TBI, such as depression, unexplained crying, anger, etc., can make it difficult for the friend to remain a friend.
- Sometimes it is just that friends have moved on in their lives. They get married; they move; they have children; they

are involved with a host of activities, or their job becomes demanding. Perhaps they now have someone in their own family that needs their attention. The point is, they have moved on to life's changes and the survivor has not.

So what should you do if you, the survivor, would like to reconnect with old friends and establish new friends?

- Old Friends — Even if married, having friends to do things with is very rewarding and it is important to give the caregiver a break. First, you must take on an attitude that says, "I can handle rejection and I will become an initiator." Start out by trying to re-connect with old friends that you haven't seen for awhile and that you think you would like to see. You will know soon enough if they are interested or not. Remember, rejection is OK.

- Facebook   Many people in your circumstances have found friendship on Facebook. Friends on Facebook do not provide the same type of friendship as an in-person friend, but it may be a good supplement. You can accomplish the same thing by participating in a stroke chat site.

- Support Groups   Another way to meet new friends is to join a support group. I have talked about the value of a support group in previous chapters. Invite someone from the group to have lunch, or better yet, start a once a week lunch group. You get to pick the people that you think might be interested.

- Class   Take a class in an adult night program that you can handle and would interest you. It is another opportunity to meet new people. The same can happen at a house of worship if you are so inclined.

- Get
  involved

  The main message here is to get out and take the initiative. Don't wait for people to contact you. The more you get involved with community groups and in groups with other stroke or TBI survivors, the more you can expand your social life.

Chapter 21: Driving After a Brain Injury

Linda is now driving after she has recovered from her stroke. She still has cognitive problems and judgment is somewhat impaired. Her family and friends have advised her not to drive, but she feels she is capable and cherishes her independence. She has promised not to drive on the highways or to drive at night. She has not had an accident since driving for the past few months, but she has hit a curb which caused a flat tire.

Driving after a stroke or traumatic brain injury is a major concern both for the survivor and for family and friends. Are there many brain injured people out there that are driving that should not be behind the wheel? I asked Beth Rolland, a driving rehabilitation specialist at the Driving Center of Kessler Institute of Rehabilitation in Saddle Brook, New Jersey, that very question.

She states, "Absolutely. I think there are many survivors who just return to driving either against medical advice, or because a doctor has not properly advised them not to drive. There are also survivors whose families pressure them to return to driving and do not understand that there are cognitive or visual deficits that cause a real danger." Beth adds, "As a driving specialist, however, my goal is to get people who have suffered a brain injury, back driving safely again."

Linda drives, not only because she thinks she is "fine to drive," but she lives alone and needs to drive to get groceries and to go various places in her community such as the hair dresser, pharmacy, the bank, etc. Others need to get to work, pick up the kids from school, go to school themselves, etc.

When Beth Rolland starts with a survivor wanting to drive, she cites several typical problems that might be present.

- Not taking the time to properly check for traffic before turning or entering a road.
- Cutting people off because they are not judging space or speed properly.

- Difficulty adjusting to something unexpected on the road, such as a construction zone or an abnormal traffic pattern.
- Slow processing speed leading to hesitation and slowness, or driving too fast without realizing it.
- Driving with attention to close to the front of the car instead of looking down the road. This results in difficulty avoiding hazards and obstructions.
- Some clients have visual problems as well. These include deficits concerning distance, coordination of sight between the the two eyes, and deficits seeing side to side. If these problems cannot be solved by an Ophthalmologist, then a driving center cannot help and the survivor should not drive.
- Some clients have physical deficits on the right side of the body and must learn to use a left side break and gas pedal.

Often survivors are not aware that it is dangerous for them to be on the road. The American Stroke Association has published a pamphlet entitled

Let's Talk About Driving After Stroke. It lists warning signs that tell you either not to drive or to get tested by a driving rehabilitation specialist. The pamphlet applies equally to TBI survivors.

- Drives too fast or too slow for road conditions or posted speeds
- Needs help or instructions from passengers
- Doesn't observe signs or signals
- Makes slow or poor distance decisions
- Gets easily frustrated or confused
- Often gets lost, even in familiar areas
- Has accidents or close calls
- Drifts across lane markings into other lanes

There is also an issue with liability. In most states, the law requires that the patient obtain medical clearance after a stroke or TBI. This must be in writing from a doctor, driving specialist, or the Motor Vehicle Department. If this is not done, the survivor is subject to a lawsuit in case of an accident.

So what should you do to be sure it is safe to drive after stroke or TBI?

Get the advice of your doctor. He or she has insight as to your ability and your deficiencies. You will be getting a professional and objective opinion based on experience.

Have your driving tested which will include a visual and behind the wheel evaluation. The instructor will test for cognitive abilities, reaction time, and judgment. Call the closest rehabilitation hospital as they often offer such programs. You can also call your local motor vehicle department to find a driving center.

Ask your family and friends if they have noticed changes in your driving. You must remember that driving a car requires multi-tasking and is usually more difficult for someone with a brain injury.

Beth Rolland emphasizes that more attention needs to be paid to get dangerous drivers who have suffered a brain injury off the road. "Doctors need to take the lead in advising survivors to contact a Driver Rehabilitation center before they drive. Health insurance companies need to understand driving rehabilitation and cover it as a medically necessary service."

She believes that survivors would use this service if it was paid for. And there should be better transportation options especially for people who live in the suburbs where public transportation may not be available.

Part IV: Research and Recovery

Chapter 22: Stem Cell Research

I know that talking about anything to do with stem cell research is a slippery slope. Many object to embryonic stem cell research, usually based on religious belief. However, there is much being done with adult stem cells taken from bone marrow and with new born umbilical cords.

I have been tracking stem cell research as it pertains to brain injury for the last five years. In March, 2010, I wrote an article for strokenetwork.org about progress being made using stem cells to help stroke survivors. I found many studies being done using rats and other animals. Most of the studies centered on safety rather than direct reversal of stroke related disabilities. The sources that I used agree that there is no stem cell treatment now (March, 2010) that has proven to improve or reverse the disabilities as a result of a stroke.

I had interviewed three doctors and researched several studies for my March, 2010 article, and recently I decided to find out what progress has been made since I wrote that article about two and a half years ago. I made every effort to re-interview each of the three that I had interviewed for the first article. I was only able to contact two of them. In the 2010 article:

Dr. Keith Muir, a neurologist and researcher at Southern General Hospital in Glasgow, Scotland, was in the middle of a safety study which eventually would lead to injecting stem cells into the brain with the hope of re-instituting brain connections lost from the stroke.

Dr. Douglas Kondziolka, a neurological surgeon at the University of Pittsburgh said, in 2010, that he knew of no stem cell studies that were using humans.

I asked these two doctors for an update.

"I know there are many stem cell studies related to stroke being done using rats and other animals, but are there now studies taking place using human stroke survivors? And how close is the medical community to reversing or minimizing the disabilities caused by a stroke?"

Dr. Muir told me about a study that he is currently heading called PISCES (Pilot Investigation of Stem Cells in Stroke). For the study, researchers are using twelve men, all over age sixty with moderate to severe neurological impairments as a result of a stroke, with four different doses of stem cell treatment. So far, all six patients who have received the stem cells have shown some promising improvements with no adverse side effects. Dr. Muir stated, "We remain pleased and encouraged by the data emerging from the PISCES study to date." Dr. Muir emphasizes, however, "this study is primarily about safety and although we are looking at function as well, functional benefit from stem cell treatment will require a second phase study. We anticipate treating the next three patents in August or September, and if all goes well, the final three patients will be treated by the middle of 2013. If there are no safety issues, we must then design a study that focuses on neurological effects of stem cell implantation."

When Dr. Muir read the draft of this chapter he told me that "researchers are very conscious of how long it takes to undertake properly conducted trials, and the speed with which these happen is influenced by many factors including trial design, regulatory oversight, trial size, and complexity. Test results are often difficult to interpret and it is quite possible that we ultimately find that there is insufficient benefit from this type of intervention to justify the risk. Anyone involved in stroke research over the past twenty years will be familiar with the many drug treatments that sounded very promising based on animal research but proved to be ineffective or harmful in humans." Dr. Muir concluded "I think a ten year time frame is probably a short time scale to expect us to test most of the cell therapies given the complexity of the issues."

Dr. Kondziolka and his team are also currently conducting an on-going human stem cell study at the University of Pittsburgh and Stanford University sponsored by SanBio Inc. The study will enroll eighteen patients that are between six months and thirty six months post ischemic stroke. It will involve a neurological procedure to administer stem cells directly into the brain. There will then be eight follow-up visits over a two year period to assess safety, but while safety is the goal, tests to assess motor, sensory, and cognitive ability will also be performed.

I found other studies in various stages of development, as well. In a February, 2012 article, two small studies in India have been concluded where patients have regained some of their lost abilities after receiving stem cells intravenously. I must caution our readers as I did in my 2010 article, that studies in other countries often do not have a control group to compare the treated group. You can read about these two studies by using Google: "Stem Cell Therapy Shows Promise for Stroke," by Maureen Salamon.

Another study is underway involving 140 patients. The study is sponsored by Althersys and will use their patented MultiStem, manufactured from human stem cells obtained from human bone marrow. This study is to be concluded by November, 2014. To read about this study, go to Google: Althersys Medcity News/ stroke.

Conclusion: There are many variables involved in stem cell research and each has to be tested: length of time post stroke, severity of disability, type of stem cells used, dosage amounts, timing of dosage, how the dose is administered, age of patient, and safety.

No study that I read, and neither of the doctors that I communicated with, could say how close they are to being able to reverse the symptoms of a stroke because there is much more research to be done. In the many studies that I researched, there seemed to be a great deal of optimism for the future, but that future could be ten to fifteen years or more away.

I intend to keep a close eye on these studies and the development of stem cell treatment for stroke survivors. I will write another article for strokenetwork.org in 2015 with an update.

Chapter 23: New Drugs on the Horizon

After suffering a stroke, many survivors are prescribed medications to help moderate resulting conditions. Warfarin and Plavix and other anti-clotting drugs, Trileptol and other anti-seizure drugs, and Botox for relieving spasticity, are examples. There are also new drugs on the horizon that may be beneficial in the future.

<u>MW151 and MW189</u>: In animal studies, these drugs have shown promise in prevention of cognitive damage after a stroke or traumatic brain injury by reducing brain inflammation. In a study with mice, Dr. Mark Wainright, professor of pediatric neurology at Northwestern's Feinberg School of Medicine and a physician at the Ann & Robert H. Lurie Children's Hospital in Chicago, showed that given MW151 between three and six hours after a stroke (or TBI), inflammation was prevented or reduced which in turn reduced damage to the brain. Dr. Wainright states, "If you took a drug like this after a TBI or stroke, you could possibly prevent the long-term complications of that injury including the risk of seizures, cognitive impairment, and, perhaps, mental health issues." (The Challenge: The Brain Injury Association of America, summer, 2012.) Studies using MW151 and MW189 are still in the early stages, so it is up to the reader to follow the progress of on-going and future studies.

Tissue Plasminogen Activator (t-PA): This is not a new drug. It has been used for many years to treat stroke patients who had an ischemic (clot) stroke, but I include t-PA in this article because it has the same goal as MW151, that is to reduce the negative impact of the stroke. For most patients, it is only effective if given intravenously or directly into an artery within the first three or four hours following stroke onset. The drug is designed as a "clot buster" freeing the blocked artery and restoring blood flow and oxygen to the brain to reduce damage. This differs from MW151 and MW189. Where MW151 works on the central nervous system, t-PA breaks up the clot in the affected artery.

I received an e-mail from Dr. Martin Watterson also from Northwestern University Medical School, and Dr. Cesar V. Borlongan, a medical researcher at the University of South Florida, in which they clarified the difference between t-PA and MW151. Whereas t-PA simply reopens the artery, it does not address secondary cell death that occurs after the stroke. MW151 reduces inflammation to the central nervous system which can continue days, weeks, months, or even years after the stroke. MW151 creates healthy neuroprotective properties and a wide therapeutic window that t-PA does not. Dr. Watterson is collaborating with Dr. Wainwright on one stroke model study and with Dr. Borlongan on another study on the use of drugs in conjunction with stem cell transplantation.

Metformin: This is not a new drug. It has been used for years to treat type 2 diabetes. But what is new, is that the drug now is being studied for repairing brain damage after a stroke or TBI. Canadian scientists state, " When we tested the drug in lab mice we found that mice given daily doses of Metforin for two or three weeks had increased brain cell growth and outperformed untreated mice in learning and memory experiments." This drug has an advantage. When studies begin with humans, the safety factor, which often delays human studies, has already been proven as it has been used for type 2 diabetes safely for many years. (from an article by Lisa Hurwitz, The Challenge: The Brain Injury Association of America, (Summer, 2012.) Once again, research is in the early stages and it is up to the reader to follow the progress of on-going and future studies.

Etanercept: This drug is only being used for stroke treatment at the Institute of Neurological Recovery (INR) in California. One can find several successful studies and endorsements for Etanercept claiming that stroke impairments, both motor control and cognition, can be radically improved. INR's web-site also has numerous videos showing subjects with great improvement ten minutes after being injected with Etanercept in the spinal area. You might also recognize this drug from golfer Phil Michelson's ad for Enbrel which is for psoriatic arthritis and is a brand name for Etanercept. The problem is that none of the studies that I found were published in any reputable journal or publication. A second problem is that there are many blogs calling the company a sham. In fairness, I think the reader should use caution with this company and its use of Etanercept. My guess is that the company will either disappear or the medical community will get on board and conduct scientific tests on Etanercept.

Chapter 24: Transcranial Magnetic Stimulation

First, some definitions:

Transcranial Magnetic Stimulation (TMS) is a non-invasive procedure using electromagnetic induction to stimulate specific areas of the brain. An electromagnet device is placed over a specific area of the skull where short pulses are administered which easily pass through the skull.

Repetitive Transcranial Magnetic Stimulation (rTMS) is a variation of TMS that involves multiple stimulations delivered at a specific frequency for a specific duration. Most studies completed or in progress that consider TMS as a treatment are with this method of TMS.

Repetitive Transcranial Magnetic Stimulation (rTMS) does show promise for stroke and rehabilitation. Although it is not yet approved by the FDA as a treatment for stroke, several studies show positive results in improving motor skills, speech, and cognition. On-going studies being conducted by Dr. Carolynn Patten, a neurologist (PhD) and physical therapist, and Dr. William Triggs, a neurologist, both researchers at the University of Florida and VA Brain Rehabilitation Research Center in Gainesville, Florida, are investigating the effects of rTMS on motor dysfunction in adults after stroke.

I contacted Dr. Patten via e-mail. She stated, "rTMS involves multiple stimulations, delivered at a specific frequency for a specific duration. Repetitive TMS modulates (alters) the excitability of the brain. Low frequency stimulation inhibits brain activity, meaning it makes the brain less easy to activate. High frequency stimulation excites brain activity making it easier to activate and makes the brain more responsive. Also, rTMS involves focal areas of the brain rather than the entire brain." By adjusting the excitability in various parts of the brain, information can be obtained about the roles of different regions of the brain.

In an e-mail that I received from Dr. Triggs, he stated, "rTMS as a treatment for stroke has potential, particularly when combined with physical and occupational therapy. However, more double blind studies using larger populations are needed before a definite conclusion can be reached."

Researchers Dr. Godfried Schlang, Dr. Vijay Renga, and Dr. Dinesh Nair, affiliated with the Department of Neurology, Beth Israel Deaconess Medical Center and Harvard Medical School, Boston, Massachusetts, found positive results with TMS including improved movement of affected limbs and improved cognitive ability without damage to brain tissue. In an article published in Neurology Review, December, 2008, the authors stated, "TMS has great potential because it is easy to implement, it is safe, and it is non-invasive. If greater studies duplicate the pilot studies being done, TMS will become an important therapy in treating stroke disabilities."

Conclusion: rTMS to improve or repair disabilities caused by stroke have shown promise. Various studies are being conducted using various delivery techniques and with different goals. The over-all objective is to reduce impairments and disability post stroke. These disabilities include limb movement and strength, swallowing (dysphagia), aphasia, and other cognitive impairments. All of the studies include the warning that research studies are ongoing, and although there is reason for optimism, it is too early to claim that rTMS is effective for stroke symptoms.

The researchers must consider:
Safety in conducting the studies.
The frequency of the stimulation to be delivered.
The hemisphere (left vs. right), and the specific area of the brain that rTMS is to be delivered. (For example targeted areas may be the area of the brain controlling speech, or visual, or motor skills).

Dr. Patten emphasizes this point. "While we have not cracked the code, there is reason for optimism. There is a lot of work to be done. I hope that people who have experienced stroke will remain open to the idea, and that their health care providers will remain open to the idea so that all the labs investigating rTMS are able to do their studies and collectively we are able to advance knowledge and improve stroke rehabilitation."

Chapter 25: Tendon Transfer Surgery for Foot Drop, Clenched Fist, and Paralysis

After a stroke or TBI, some survivors experience paralysis of one arm along with a clenched fist. If a nerve is injured preventing that nerve from sending signals to a muscle or muscles, the result is paralysis and loss of muscle function. This results in virtually no use of the affected arm and hand, and, in some cases discomfort. When a near-by tendon is not affected, it may be possible to transfer a functional tendon from its original attachment to a new attachment restoring some use to the non functioning area.

Tendon Transfer Hand Surgery

What exactly is hand tendon transfer surgery? Below the elbow, there are between forty and fifty muscles. When a muscle or muscles are neurologically destroyed due to stroke, they can no longer signal the arm or hand to function. There are three major nerves in the hand: the ulnar nerve, the radial nerve, and the median nerve. When any of these are injured or destroyed, paralysis, loss of feeling, and clenched fist is the result.

How successful is hand tendon surgery? Hand tendon transfer may be successful in restoring some function to the hand or arm. In a 2008 study in the Netherlands (LC Heijnen et. al.) six patients were followed who had hand tendon transfer surgery for clenched fist. After the surgery, all six could passively open their hands in a resting position, and some flexible movement was gained in each case. There were no complications after nineteen months and all six patients were still able to keep their hands open. There was also permanent improvement in pain reduction and hygiene.

I asked Dr. Andrew Elkwood how much success he has had doing this surgery. Dr. Elkwood practices plastic surgery at the Plastic Surgery Center in Shrewsbury, New Jersey. He is considered an expert in nerve reconstruction surgery for patients who have lost the use of a limb due to nerve damage. He has also been featured on the T.V. show, "The Doctors." Dr. Elkwood was reluctant to profile what a good tendon transfer surgical candidate looked like because diagnosis depends on so many factors, such as how many nerves and or muscles are damaged, and to what degree they are damaged. He stated, "I like to examine, evaluate, and then give my assessment as to the expected results of surgery."

Dr. Elkwood also told me that the hand is more difficult than the arm to restore. After surgery, even if function cannot be restored, at the very least, the patient will be able to open the hand. "No one gains 100% of function but there are some who show great improvement, some who cannot be helped at all, and many who fall in between these two categories."

Tendon Transfer Surgery for Foot Drop:

Seven years ago, Sandy Smethers, a stroke survivor that I was mentoring (and still am), was recommended by a neurologist to consider tendon transfer for her drop foot. We went to Pennsylvania University Hospital in Philadelphia to see Dr. Maryann Keenan, an orthopedic surgeon. Dr. Keenan recommended tendon transfer surgery and she performed it shortly after our visit. Sandy's surgery was only partly successful. Her foot was restored to a more normal position, but she still requires a brace and walks with a considerable limp. However, her balance improved and she now walks without a cane,

Foot drop, or drop foot, has many causes and varied symptoms. A stroke or TBI survivor who has foot drop has difficulty lifting the front of the foot. As a result, the survivor may drag the affected foot on the ground making walking difficult. Many survivors will trip with a drop foot. To compensate, those affected may raise the thigh unusually high, and may swing the affected foot out to the side to avoid lifting the thigh upward. The immediate aid is to wear a brace from the upper calf, down past the ankle extending under the entire foot. This will keep the foot in a normal position.

I was able to reach podiatric foot and ankle surgeon, Dr. Lawrence DiDomenico by telephone.

Dr. DiDomenico is a podiatric physician and surgeon at the Ankle and Footcare Center in Youngstown, Ohio. Dr. DiDomenico stated, "with classic foot drop, the common peroneal nerve is affected and leads to anterior and lateral (front and outside muscles of the leg) muscle group weakness, which controls the foot." Diagnosis of the cause is imperative as that will determine the course of treatment. Dr. DiDomenico told me that treatment options for foot drop include prescribing a brace, gait training, physical therapy, and tendon transfer surgery.

You, as a patient must discuss these options with your podiatric surgeon or orthopedic surgeon. But once the diagnosis calls for tendon transfer, the tendon transfer surgery is performed with the goal of restoring the function of the foot and ankle to a more normal anatomical alignment so that the patient can walk on the sole of the foot with the heel touching the ground, improving gait and balance when walking in a shoe and without a brace.

Dr. DiDomenico told me that the large majority of tendon transfers for foot drop are done by podiatric surgeons and orthopedic surgeons that have an expertise and interest in foot and ankle surgery. "The surgery involves rerouting the posterior tibial tendon, a tendon that functions well from the back of the leg, and transferring it to the front of the leg and connecting it to the top of the foot. This compensates for the loss of muscle function in the front of the leg as a result of the stroke. Although 100% improvement is not expected, between 40% and 50% is typical."

Appendix I: Stroke Care in Europe

As a volunteer for the Brain Injury Association of New Jersey, I have been a Mentor for stroke survivors for several years. I am always looking for new ideas on how to help stroke survivors and caregivers. When planning a seven week trip to Europe, I included a plan to investigate stroke care in at least one other country.

While in the Czech Republic, I visited the Stroke Unit at Charles University Hospital in Prague. Upon my return, I did some research on stroke care in other countries in Europe. Like in the United States, stroke is the third leading cause of death in Europe, behind heart disease and cancer. Also, as in the US, there is not enough attention paid to stroke, frustrating neurologists and hospitals that serve stroke patients.

Treatment of stroke patients in Europe is similar to treatment in the US with very few differences.

Typically, in the US, when a patient arrives in a hospital after a stroke, that patient undergoes a rapid evaluation followed by critical care treatment. The patient stays in that hospital until he is out of danger.

At that time the patient is transferred to a rehabilitation hospital where physical, occupational, and speech therapy takes place until he is released. The patient then continues that therapy on an outpatient basis for an undetermined length of time. (in the US it is often determined by medical insurance coverage.)

I interviewed Dr. Ctirad Lakomy, a Neurologist in the Neurointensive Care Unit of Charles University Hospital in Prague, (Department of Neurology of the First Faculty of Medicine and General Teaching Hospital, Charles University in Prague) about stroke care in the Czech Republic and in Europe.

Q: In both the US and the Czech Republic, stroke is the third leading cause of death and the leading cause of disability. What is the medical community doing to combat the problem?

A: I would like to see more done. There are regular media campaigns to educate people regarding stroke warning signs and stroke prevention. This includes pamphlets and bulletins sent to doctors and hospitals. We do not have a national magazine or newsletters which would be a real help to stroke survivors.

Q: A recent study revealed that 20% of adults in the US smoke and 33% of Czech adults smoke. Do you consider that significant?

A: That number does not surprise me. But of course it is very high and contributes to incidence of stroke. People in both countries must take the danger of smoking more seriously.

Q: Please describe the process or sequence for treatment once a stroke patient enters your hospital.

A: Time is important so testing for diagnosis is most important. We do immediate clinical and laboratory screening which means a CT Scan (Computed Tomography), an angiogram to measure blood flow to the brain, an ultra sound of the carotid arteries, a trans cranial color coded sonography which measures the velocity of blood flow through the brain's blood vessels, and trembolysi (administering clot busting medication) when called for. The patient then is monitored closely until they are ready for the rehabilitation stage.

Q: The Czech Republic has socialized medicine. Is this good or bad?

A: I don't like it. It puts a financial strain on hospitals because stroke patients stay hospitalized longer than most other patients. I also believe that the system in general makes people more passive about their health care. Also, in our country, doctors are paid poorly which discourages many talented young people from becoming doctors.

Q: How many stroke centers are there in the Czech Republic?

A: There are 50 registered centers capable of administering clot busting drugs. The problem is that some outlying areas are without a stroke unit.

This is a serious concern throughout the medical community in the Czech Republic. According to Dr. R. Herzig, et. al., in a study done from the medical faculty at Palacky University in Olomouc, Czech Republic, only 75% of the Czech

Districts are covered by a stroke unit. This study was done because the medical community is trying to improve that situation.

I wanted to find out if there were new treatments in Europe that we in the US could benefit from so I asked Dr. Lakomy if he knew of any treatment in Europe that could benefit patients in the United States. Dr. Lakomy told me that there is great cooperation between the European Union countries, Canada, and the US. All of these countries are continuously sharing their latest developments through international conferences, articles in journals, joint studies, and shared seminars.

So what do European and American doctors advise about stroke? First, don't wait to have a stroke before you act. Prevention is key. There is a website in Europe called http://www.safestroke.org. It stands for Stroke Alliance for Europe and it is totally in English. On the site's home page, it states that 80% of all strokes are preventable by not smoking, drinking in moderation, and having regular exams to be sure blood pressure, cholesterol, triglycerides, and blood sugar are normal.

Second, know the hospital closest to you that has emergency stroke care available twenty four hours a day. Be sure they have the proper evaluation equipment and are capable of administering clot busting drugs.

And third, do not ignore the warning signs of a stroke. The sooner you get to the hospital the better chance you have for survival and recovery.

Appendix II: A Partial List of Helpful Web sites and Free Magazines

Web-sites

www.americanheart.org
www.nih.gov
www.ninds.nih.gov
www.clinicaltrials.gov
www.curebraindisease.org
www.strokeassociation.org
www.nationalstrokeassociation.org
www.strokesafe.org
www.safestroke.org
www.biaa.org
www.stroke.org
www.aan.com/patients (neurology)
www.thefamilycaregiver.org
www.aphasia.org
www.aphasia.net
www.asha.org (for aphasia)

www.academyofaphasia.org
www.apraxia-kids.org
www.alexiafoundation.org
www.wellspouse.org

Appendix III: Primary Stroke Centers

Stroke is the third leading cause of death and the leading cause of disability. It is important to know where the closest qualified Primary Stroke Center is located. Research studies show that stroke survivors treated at a PSC hospital have the best chance of recovery and survival. These PSC hospitals are certified by The Joint Commission. I asked Katrina Maule, Stroke Program Coordinator at Lancaster General Hospital, Lancaster, Pennsylvania, to explain The Joint Commission.

She said, "The Joint Commission is an independent, not-for-profit organization established more than 50 years ago. They are governed by a board that includes physicians, nurses, and consumers. The Joint Commission sets the standards by which health care quality is measured in America and around the world. It evaluates the quality and safety of care for more than 17,000 health care organizations."

In a May, 2010, the American Stroke Association conducted a study to determine whether people were aware of the PSC hospitals in the area where they live. The results were published in the May/June 2010 issue of Stroke Connection Magazine (P. 7).

The A.S.A. surveyed 1,000 people from the general public and 460 stroke survivors and caregivers. 58% of the general population and 45% of the survivors and caregivers did not know if their closest hospital was a PSC. These results indicate that there is a need to educate people as to where to go in the event of a stroke.

How exactly does a Primary Stroke Center qualify for certification by The Joint Commission? Certification is based on the recommendations of the Brain Attack Coalition. In order to receive Primary Stroke Care status, a hospital must accomplish the following within a three hour period:

- Transport the patient to the hospital
- Perform a full evaluation by a neurologist

- Obtain and read a CT scan of the brain
- Draw blood, analyze it, and report the results
- Deliver appropriate treatment

The most common barrier preventing a patient from getting emergency treatment is delayed diagnosis in a busy emergency room. That is a major reason to go to a Primary Stroke Center hospital.

In order to provide the five major accomplishments listed above, the Brain Attack Coalition recommends that PSC hospitals have round the clock neurological services including a physician with expertise in interpreting CT scan and immediate use of CT scanners. The hospital must have an acute stroke team including a physician and at least one other health-care professional available around the clock.

The hospital must provide training to rescue squads, emergency room staff, and to doctors, and nurses in a designated stroke unit with a stroke center director. The hospital also must follow long term stroke treatment outcomes and design quality improvement activities for the patient.

Katrina Maule added that it takes four months of compliance before a hospital can be certified. The Joint Commission awards certification for one year for those hospitals that demonstrate they have met these requirements. This is followed by an on-site review by the Joint Commission every two years.

To find a Primary Stroke Center near you:

- Go to www.strokeassociation.org
- Click on "Find Stroke Care Near You"
- Fill out your zip code
- Select a hospital

About the author:

Walter Kilcullen is a retired guidance counselor from Morris Knolls High School, Rockaway, New Jersey. He has been a mentor for stroke and traumatic brain injury survivors for the past twelve years. He lives in Allamuchy, New Jersey with his wife Susan